WHAT IS CRPS?
A HELPFUL GUIDE TO TEACH CHILDREN ABOUT
COMPLEX REGIONAL PAIN SYNDROME (CRPS)
Volume III

Alaa Abd-Elsayed M.D., MPH, FASA and Eric M. Phillips

All rights are preserved for publisher, The MG Academy LLC. No part of this book may be reproduced or transmitted in any form or by any means electronic or mechanical including photocopying, recording or by any information storage and retrieval system without permission in writing from the copyright owner, The MG Academy LLC.

First edition, 2020 - Volume III

ISBN: 9798585980954

Other books published by authors:

Alaa Abd-Elsayed

- Chronic Pain: The Patient and Family Journey
- If the Savior is not Safe, How Can He Save?
- Pain: A Review Guide
- Infusion Therapy for Pain, Headache and Related Conditions
- Complex Regional Pain Syndrome (CRPS): Patients' Perspective of Living in Chronic Pain: Volume 1
- Complex Regional Pain Syndrome (CRPS): Patients' Perspective of Living in Chronic Pain: Volume 1-Picture eBook
- Complex Regional Pain Syndrome (CRPS): Patients' Perspective of Living in Chronic Pain: Volume II
- Complex Regional Pain Syndrome (CRPS): A Patients' Picture eBook Guide: Volume II

Eric M. Phillips

- Complex Regional Pain Syndrome (CRPS): Patients' Perspective of Living in Chronic Pain: Volume 1
- Complex Regional Pain Syndrome (CRPS): Patients' Perspective of Living in Chronic Pain: Volume 1-Picture eBook

- Don't Diet: Change Your Eating Habits - Proper Eating for Good Health
- Complex Regional Pain Syncrome (CRPS): Patients' Perspective of Living in Chronic Pain: Volume II
- Complex Regional Pain Syndrome (CRPS): A Patients' Picture eBook Guide: Volume II

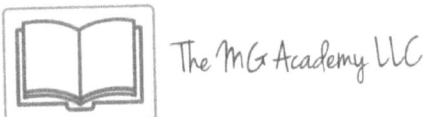

Dedication

To my parents, my wife and my two beautiful kids Maro and George.

To all CRPS patients.

Alaa Abd-Elsayed

Dedication

To my loving parents, Janet and my late father Leonard (Lenny) for all their love, and support.

To my beautiful and supportive wife Mercedes, her three children and her grandson.

To my mentor, teacher and greatest friend the late Doctor Hooshang Hooshmand.

To all CRPS patients worldwide.

Eric M. Phillips

TABLE OF CONTENTS

PREFACE
Alaa Abd-Elsayed, MD, MPH and Eric M. Phillips
Page 1

INTRODUCTION
Alaa Abd-Elsayed, MD, MPH, and Eric M. Phillips
Page 2

WHAT IS CRPS? INTRODUCTION
Alaa Abd-Elsayed, MD, MPH and Eric M. Phillips
Page 3

WHAT IS CRPS?
Page 6

SYMPTOMS OF CRPS
Page 8

STAGES OF CRPS
Page 11

WHAT IS THE SYMPATHETIC NERVOUS SYSTEM?
Page 13

TEST TO DIAGNOSE CRPS
Page 15

WHAT IS A NERVE BLOCK?
Page 18

TYPES OF NERVE BLOCKS
Page 20

CRPS AFFECTS EVERYONE DIFFERENTLY
Page 23

WHO CAN DEVELOP CRPS?
Page 26

HOW MANY YEARS HAS CRPS BEEN AROUND FOR?
Page 28

WHY IS YOUR LOVED ONE ALWAYS IN PAIN?
Page 31

WHY YOUR LOVED ONE MAY USE A WHEELCHAIR, CRUTCHES, CANE OR BRACES
Page 35

WHY YOUR LOVED ONE MAY HAVE A DEFORMED LIMB?
Page 38

CRPS CHANGES A PERSON'S LIFE
Page 40

CONCLUSION
Page 44

CRPS AWARENESS
Page 47

CRPS INFORMATION
Page 49

PREFACE

Complex regional pain syndrome (CRPS) is a very serious condition and dealing with it otherwise is not wise. Unfortunately, there is a huge lack of knowledge even among health care providers about the seriousness of this condition and what it can lead to if not managed quickly and aggressively. Early and aggressive management can lead to control and even cure of the pain, but lack of diagnosis and not understanding the urgency of treating this condition can lead to a worsening of pain with associated depression, anxiety, limb atrophy, amputation, and potential suicide.

Together we have I authored volume I and volume II of this book to share the stories of patients suffering from CRPS. This third volume of this book will focus on teaching children about what CRPS is. CRPS affects not just the patient, but their entire family, from their spouses to their children. Children are the ones that can have the most difficult time coping and understanding why their parent, relative, or friend is suffering from CRPS. It is vital to teach children why their parent or loved one is suffering and are not able to do things with them at time due to the pain of CRPS.

Our goal is to increase awareness of the severity of this condition. It is very important to provide support to CRPS patients and their families. It is important to help educate their children on how CRPS affects a person's life.

Alaa Abd-Elsayed, MD, MPH, FASA and Eric M. Phillips

INTRODUCTION

Alaa Abd-Elsayed, MD, MPH, FASA, and Eric M. Phillips

Complex regional pain syndrome (CRPS), is a poorly understood condition by the medical community. Many patients may suffer long before getting diagnosed or even receive proper treatment.

As we are all well aware of CRPS is a complex disease to diagnose, treat, and to understand.

CRPS is a painful disease that affects the patient physically, mentally, and emotionally. It can also affect the entire family because of the patient's pain. CRPS can disrupt the everyday living for the patient and their children. It can change the family's daily routine, missing important event for their children, and other family events. This can be stressful for the patient and the whole family.

We have created this book to help teach children about CRPS. We hope this book will help children learn and understand what their parent, relative, or friend goes through when they are suffering from CRPS.

Education about CRPS is a key for every member of the patient's family.

WHAT IS CRPS?
INTRODUCTION

Alaa Abd-Elsayed, M.D., and

Eric M. Phillips

What is CRPS? "A Helpful Guide to Teach Children About CRPS" is a helpful guide for children to learn and understand what their parent, relative, or friend is suffering from when they have CRPS.

The term CRPS stands for Complex Regional Pain Syndrome. CRPS is a disease of the sympathetic nervous system, which is our involuntary nervous system in our bodies. CRPS can develop from minor trauma (sprain ankle or wrist, etc...) or from a surgery (knee or shoulder surgery, etc...).

When one develops CRPS, their affected limb (hand/arm or foot/leg) becomes very painful. The pain a CRPS patient may feel in their limb could be a hot burning type of pain (it feels like their limb is on fire) or a feeling of an ice-cold pain (the feeling of their limb is placed in a bucket of ice). The pain they feel is felt 24-hours a day. The pain a patient feel is very painful all the time.

The best way to explain the pain is maybe you had a really bad toothache that was very painful for you to feel. Just imagine feeling that painful toothache all the time. That is what CRPS feels like. Very painful! Sometimes it may take a CRPS patient a few months to a few years to get diagnosed.

In this book, you will learn about the symptoms of CRPS and the stages of the disease, and the different treatments for CRPS.

You will also learn why your loved one who suffers from CRPS is in so much pain.

We hope you will enjoy learning about what CRPS is and understand why your parent or loved one is in so much pain.

So, kids now it's time for you to learn about CRPS from Nala the CRPS Service Dog. Have fun learning with Nala.

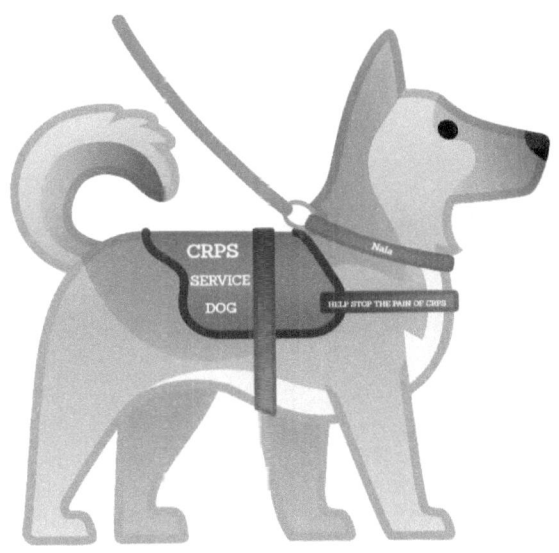

WHAT IS CRPS?

CRPS (complex regional pain syndrome) is a painful condition caused by a minor trauma either accidentally or surgically to an extremity (arm, hand, leg, or foot). Some cases of CRPS can develop after a car accident, a fall, a twisted ankle or wrist, or from surgery of the knee, shoulder, or other parts of the body. These are just some of the ways people can develop this painful condition.

There are two main symptoms of CRPS. These symptoms are a **<u>hot burning pain</u>** or an <u>ice-cold pain</u> that is felt in the affected limb. The burning pain feels like the patient's limb is on fire and the ice-cold pain feels like the affected limb is placed into a bucket of freezing cold-ice.

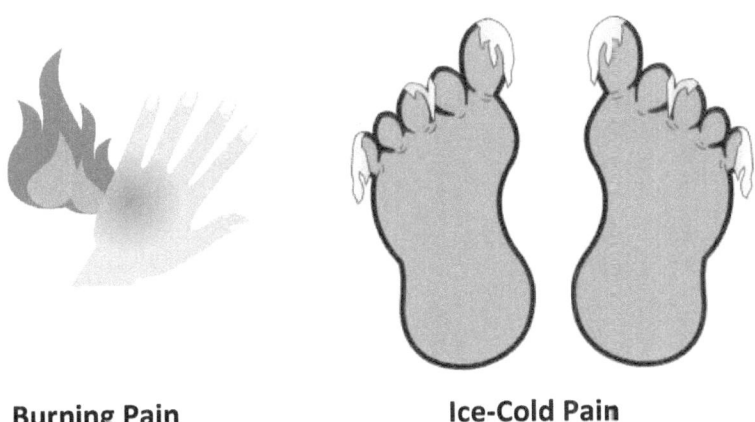

Burning Pain   Ice-Cold Pain

SYMPTOMS OF CRPS

Allodynia: This is a symptom when a patient feels pain from a non-painful-stimuli (such as a gentle breeze, bedsheets, or hair brushing against the skin) can cause pain for the patient. The slightest touch can hurt and cause more pain for the patient.

Hyperpathia: A abnormally painful reaction to a stimulus.

Atrophy: The decreased size of a body part (for example an arm/leg or hand/foot).

Edema: Swelling of a limb or digit (fingers or toes)

Nail Changes: The finger or toenails become ridged, or brittle. Patients can also have rapid nail growth.

Skin Changes: Discoloration of the skin (it can look red or blue-purple). The skin can become thin and brittle (tissue atrophy).

Hair Changes: Rapid hair growth or rapid hair loss on the affected limb.

Muscle Spasms: Sudden involuntary movement in one or more muscles in the affected limb.

Thermal Changes: Skin temperature changes. The affected limb can be either burning hot or ice-cold.

Spread of CRPS: Spread of symptoms of CRPS into another limb or another part of the body (for example the face).

STAGES OF CRPS

Stage-I: Dysfunction.

Symptoms: Hyperpathia; allodynia; muscle weakness; flexor spasms; thermal changes.

Stage-II: Dystrophy.

Symptoms: Edema; skin; hair and nail changes.

Stage-III: Atrophy.

Symptoms: Muscle atrophy; neurovascular instability; cutaneous rash or skin ulcers.

Stage-IV: Irreversible disturbance of plasticity; autonomic failure.

Symptoms: Systemic autonomic failure; visceral edema; irreversible low BP; MRSA; elephantiasis; cancer.

WHAT IS THE SYMPATHETIC NERVOUS SYSTEM?

The sympathetic nervous system is part of the autonomic nervous system, which is our involuntary nervous system. The sympathetic nervous system controls your vital signs (blood pressure, pulse, and respiration).

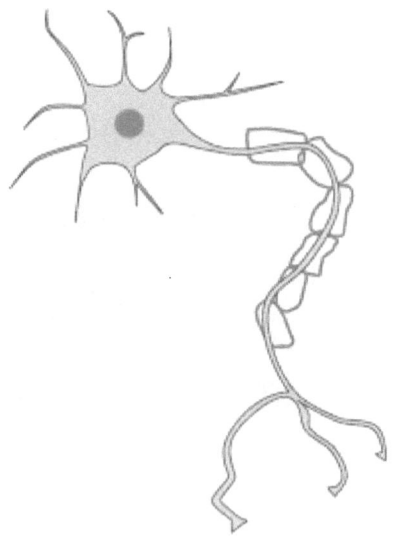

Nerve

TEST TO DIAGNOSE CRPS

There are a few tests to help with the diagnosis of CRPS.

Bone Scan: Three-phase bone scan is an imaging test to help diagnose CRPS, with the help of injecting a radioactive trace dye, to see if the patient has an increased blood flow, blood pooling, or delayed metabolism in the affected limb.

Thermography: Infrared thermal imaging (ITI) is a test that measures skin temperature differences. ITI compares the skin temperature between the affected CRPS limb and the non-affected limb. ITI creates a computerized image that shows the changes of temperature in the affected limb.

There are many other tests that may be helpful in the diagnosis of CRPS.

All these tests can be used to help with the diagnosis of CRPS. Remember no test is 100% accurate.

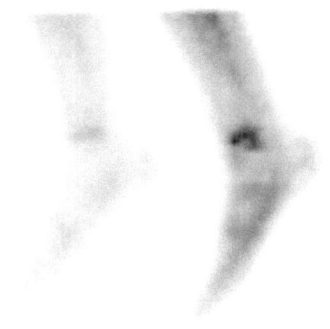

Bone Scan Image

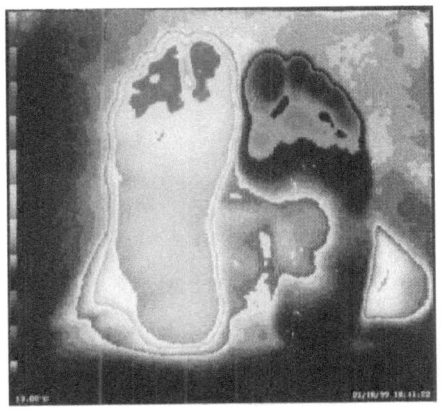

Thermography Image

WHAT IS A NERVE BLOCK?

A nerve block is a test to help a doctor diagnose CRPS. The doctor inserts a needle near the patient's spine and injects a numbing medication (anesthetic) near the sympathetic nerve. These injections have a dual purpose. They can help with a diagnosis of CRPS and it can give the patient some pain relief.

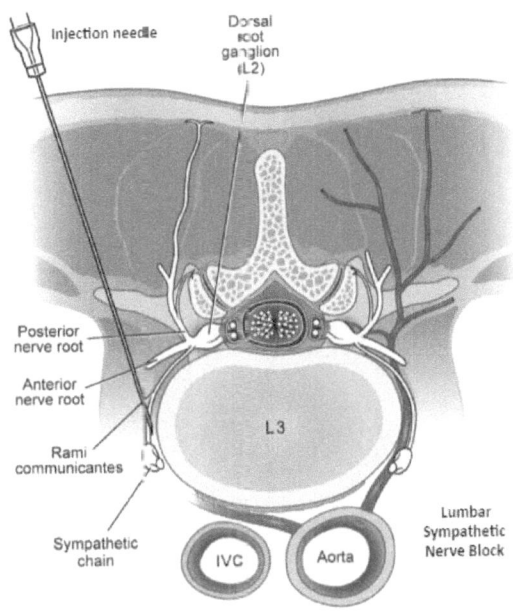

Nerve Block Image

TYPES OF NERVE BLOCKS

There are many different types of nerve blocks that may be helpful to some patients.

Sympathetic Nerve Block: This type of block is more of a diagnostic block rather than a therapeutic block for CRPS.

Epidural Block: This type of block uses a corticosteroid and it is placed in the epidural space of the spine.

Bier Block: This type of block is an intravenous regional block. During this type of block, the doctor injects a local anesthetic and other medications such as Guanethidine into the vein of the affected limb. Also, a blood-pressure cuff is placed onto the proximal part of the limb before the injection is started for about 20 to 30 minutes. This is done to prevent the loss of the medication into the systemic circulation.

Brachial Plexus Block: This type of block is used for patients with upper extremity CRPS. The location of this block can be placed in the neck, above the collarbone, or in the upper arm by the armpit. This block can be performed with a single needle or with a catheter.

These types of blocks mentioned above are performed by an anesthesiologist under the guidance of using a Fluoroscope (C-Arm), to help them guide the needle into the patient's body.

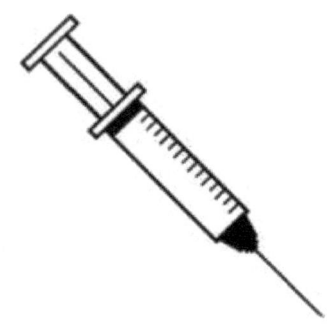

Injection Needle

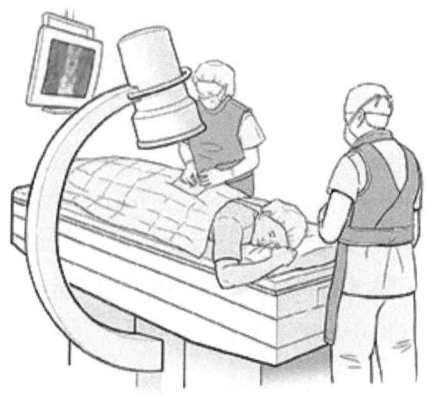

Nerve Block under Fluoroscopy Guidance

CRPS AFFECTS EVERYONE DIFFERENTLY

CRPS affects everyone differently. Some patients can have CRPS in just one limb (hand, foot, arm, or leg) or there are cases where patients may have CRPS in more than one limb or all four limbs. When a patient has it in all four limbs and other parts of the body it is called total body CRPS.

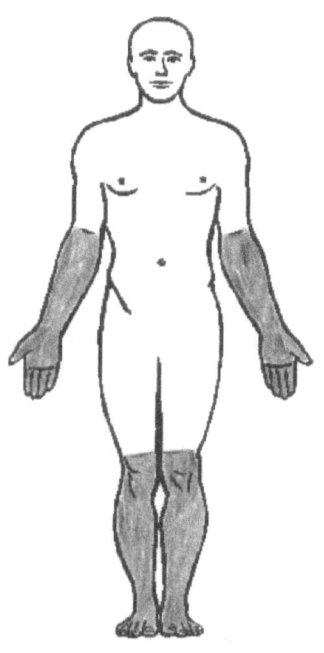

**Total Body CRPS
(All Four Limbs)**

In some cases, CRPS can start in one limb, and it can spread into another limb or other parts of the body over time. Sometimes CRPS can spread to another part of the body after having surgery or from another trauma to the body.

Each patient has a different way of coping with their CRPS pain. Some patients cope with it well and some patients have a difficult time mentally coping with the pain of CRPS.

The symptoms of CRPS can last for years to decades in some patients. Remember each case is different.

WHO CAN DEVELOP CRPS?

CRPS can happen to anyone. Men, women, and children can develop CRPS at any age. As we have mentioned earlier in the book, CRPS can develop after minor trauma or from surgery to an extremity.

Some cases of CRPS have developed after a work-related injury, crush injuries, car accidents, animal bites, slip and fall injuries, sports related injuries, and from many different types of surgery such as the knee, shoulder, carpal tunnel, and back surgery are a few different ways of developing this painful condition.

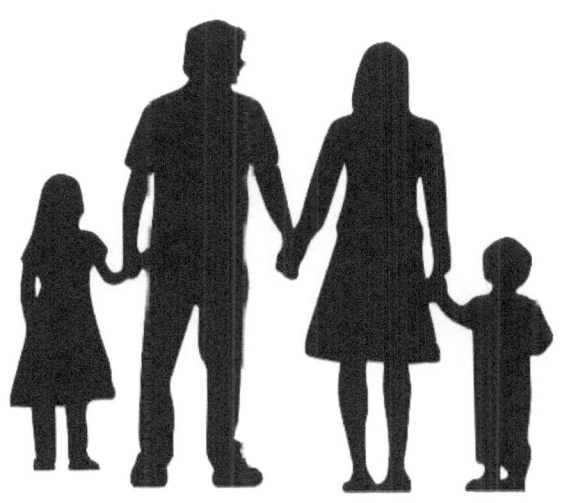

HOW MANY YEARS HAS CRPS BEEN AROUND FOR?

CRPS has been documented in the United States since 1864 (156 years). During the American Civil War, Doctor Silas Weir Mitchell the father of American neurology gave the description of causalgia (which is the original term for CRPS) in his classic article Gunshot Wounds and Other Injuries of Nerves, but it was not until 1867 when he coined the term of causalgia (CRPS) from the Greek words, "Kausos" (heat) and "algos" (pain) to describe this syndrome.

Over the years there have been many names giving to this painful condition. Other names that have been used are: reflex sympathetic dystrophy (RSD); Sudeck atrophy; reflex neurovascular dystrophy; shoulder-hand syndrome; and Algodystrophy are just a few different names used to describe CRPS. As you can see CRPS has had a long history.

When Doctor Mitchell first started to report cases of causalgia (CRPS) he saw soldiers who were wounded by gunshots during the battles of the Civil War.

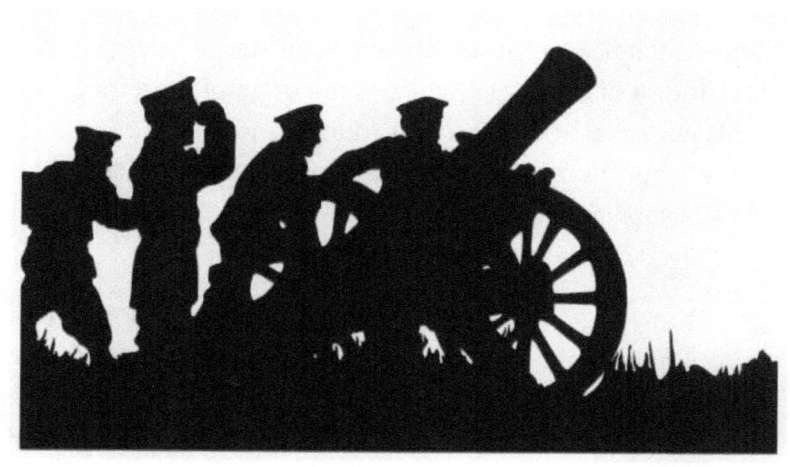

American Civil War
April 12, 1861- May 13, 1865

WHY IS YOUR LOVED ONE IS ALWAYS IN PAIN?

When your mom, dad, relative, or friend suffers from CRPS, they are always in pain. The patient's life and everyday living changes for them due to their pain.

Because your loved one is in so much pain; they might not be able to do everyday things with you like play games, play sports, or spend time going places with you, because they are in a lot of pain. You have to learn and understand that your mom, dad, relative, or friend feels bad because they are not able to do all these funs things with you due to their pain. You have to understand that they want to do all these fun things with you, but because of their pain, they cannot do it at times. They really feel bad and they just want you to understand why they cannot do things when they are in pain.

When your loved one has CRPS they are in constant pain 24-hours a day and seven days a week. Over time their affected limb becomes so painful that it cannot be touched. You may see your loved one guard (protect) their affected CRPS limb from being touched or bumped by others. Sometimes a hug can cause a CRPS patient to have more pain. It is always a good idea to ask someone who has CRPS if it is okay to give them a hug because you do not want to cause them more pain.

There are many other things that can make the pain of CRPS pain worse for your loved one. Weather changes can cause more pain for them. Sometimes hot and humid or cold and damp weather can cause a patient more pain.

Also, sometimes loud noises can cause a patient to have more pain too. Driving in a car can also give some patients more pain due to the bumpy roads, or a long ride can cause a lot of pain and discomfort for the patient.

There are times when your loved one has to go to many doctor's appointments or go to physical therapy. These appointments can be very exhausting, stressful, and painful for your loved one.

At times your loved one may be on different medications to help treat their pain and sometimes these medications may work and sometimes they do not. This is part of living with CRPS.

Sometimes your loved one may have to go for treatments like having a nerve block, to help with their pain or they may have to have surgery. These treatments and surgeries can cause your loved one a lot of stress and more pain if the treatment or surgery does not help or work for them.

Another symptom that CRPS patients may develop is depression. This is when they feel sad due to their pain. When patients feel sad, their pain may increase and they may not want to do things with their family or friends. We all should be sympathetic and understanding why they are feeling like this. The reason they may feel like this at times is due to living many years in chronic pain from the CRPS. It's not your loved one's fault. It happens to a lot of patients who suffer from CRPS.

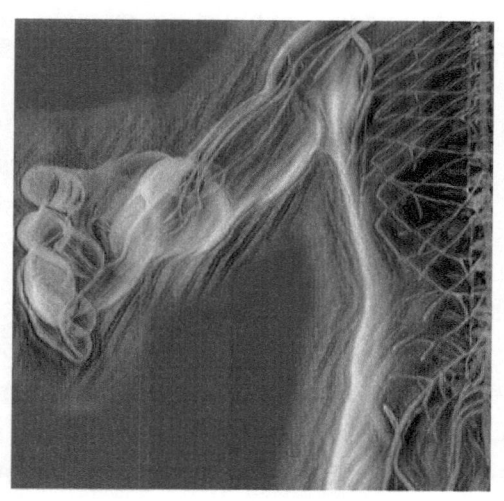

The Pain of CRPS

WHY YOUR LOVED ONE MAY USE A WHEELCHAIR, CRUTCHES, CANE, OR A BRACES

For some patients with lower limb CRPS, they may need the aid of a wheelchair, crutches, or cane to move around in the house, to go food shopping, going to a park or a zoo with you. The reason that some CRPS patients may need these devices is due to their pain or because they lost the use of the affected limb due to CRPS. These devices can help them to be more mobile in life.

For patients with upper extremity (hand, wrist arm, or should) CRPS they may need to wear some type of brace or splint on their affected upper limb. These types of braces or splints are used to help support their affected limb.

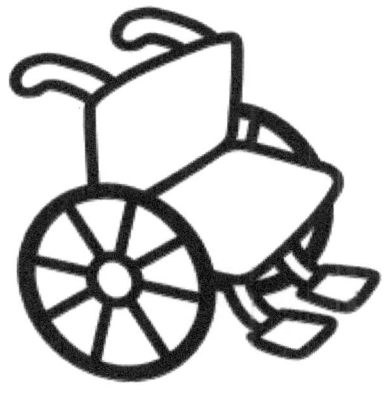
Wheelchair

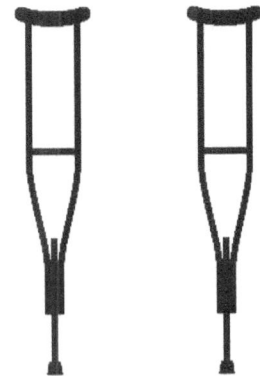
Crutches

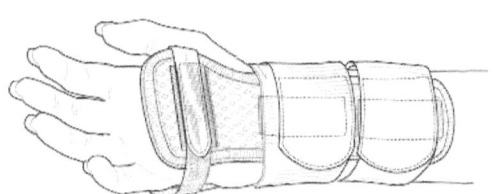
Hand Brace

WHY YOUR LOVED ONE MAY HAVE A DEFORMED LIMB?

Your loved one may suffer from a limb deformity. This is another complication seen in some CRPS patients. Some patients can develop a limb deformity (curled toes or fingers) earlier in the course of the disease. There are some patients that can develop these deformities later on in the course of their disease too, it depends on many different factors. These deformities can affect the toes, ankle, foot, fingers, hand, or wrist.

When patients develop these deformities, it can affect their walking, handwriting, and doing basic things with their hands. These deformities can also add more pain to the patient.

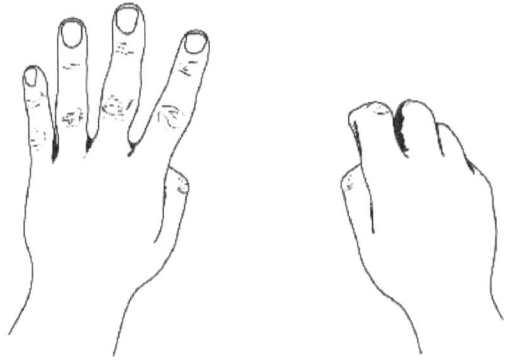

Right Hand Deformity Caused By CRPS

CRPS CHANGES A PERSON'S LIFE

CRPS is a painful condition that changes a person's life.

Your loved one may suffer from CRPS for months to many years. Unfortunately, CRPS does not only affect the patient, it also affects the whole family.

CRPS can disrupt everyday life for the whole family. CRPS changes the patient's ability to do things with and for their family.

Living with CRPS affects many aspects of a person's life from having to modify their home if they are in a wheelchair or if they need special things at home to make their life easier.

Having CRPS can change the relationships patients have with their loved ones and friends.

CRPS can also affect things when a patient is unable to go to family events and outings (birthday parties, weddings, family reunions, etc...). It can also affect doing things with their children and friends.

Remember it is not the fault of your mom, dad, relative, or friend when they are unable to do things with you and the whole family.

A helpful thing you can do for your loved ones is to ask questions about their CRPS and their pain. By asking questions it helps you learn and understand what they are going through.

This can help make your loved one feel better when they can teach you and help you understand what they are living with and what they are going through.

There are good days and bad days for some patients suffering from CRPS. Maybe on a good day your mom, dad, relative, or friend can spend a day with you to have some fun? Try to be patient with your loved one and understand how their pain affects them.

The best medicine for CRPS patients is to have their family and friends show their love and support for them. Try to be there for them during the difficult and painful times they are dealing with.

Your love and support can create a positive uplifting feeling for your loved one suffering from CRPS. This is very helpful for them. This feeling can give them a big boost in dealing with the pain of CRPS. It also gives them a feeling that they are not alone in their battle against CRPS.

Remember: "The pain of CRPS burns like an endless flame".

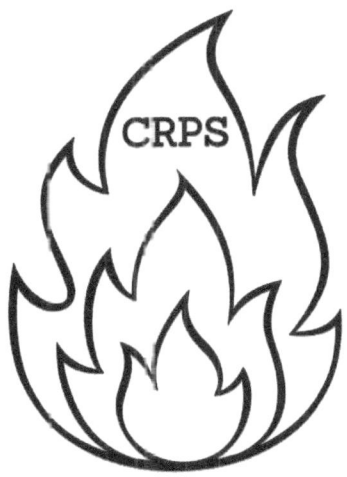

Maybe someday we can find a cure for CRPS to help put out the endless burning flame of pain.

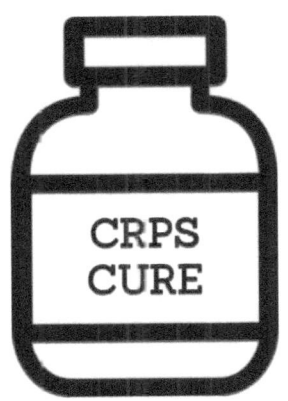

CONCLUSION

CRPS is a painful condition that affects millions of people worldwide. Patients suffer daily and, on many levels, due to their pain.

CRPS affects the whole family, and children are affected greatly.

When a patient develops CRPS, they deal with many difficult obstacles such as, getting a proper diagnosis, getting proper treatment, and receiving support from their family and friends.

When a patient is coping with CRPS, they have to adjust to the physical and emotional changes that are caused by the disease.

It is a good idea to ask your parent, relative or friend about the treatments (such as nerve blocks) and medication they have to go through and have to take to help their pain. By learning about the treatments and medications for CRPS, it will help you understand what your loved one goes through during the course of their disease.

Support for a patient living with CRPS is very important. If a patient does not have support from their family, it may cause the patient more pain and possibly depression for some patients.

Family support is vital for CRPS patients. It helps them get through their treatments and surgeries they may have to go through.

Living with CRPS is a long road for the patient, their family and friends. It's helpful for the patient when they can teach others about this painful condition.

Your loved one knows that there are times when their pain makes life difficult for you, when you want to do things with them, like play a game or go places with them.

As, you learn more about CRPS, the more you will understand why your loved one is in pain and why it may be difficult for them to do things with you.

Maybe you can find other fun things to do with your loved one when they are having a good day with their pain.

Remember the more you learn, the more you will know about CRPS. Never be afraid to ask questions. It's always fun to learn new things in life and to learn about something that affects your loved one is very important.

We hope this book has helped you learn a little bit about what CRPS is and what your loved one is dealing with daily.

CRPS AWARENESS

CRPS education and awareness are very important to patients and their family members.

By learning from your loved one who is suffering from CRPS, it will help you educate and others about CRPS. The more you learn, the more you can help spread awareness about CRPS.

Through education, awareness, and research maybe someday we can find a cure for CRPS?

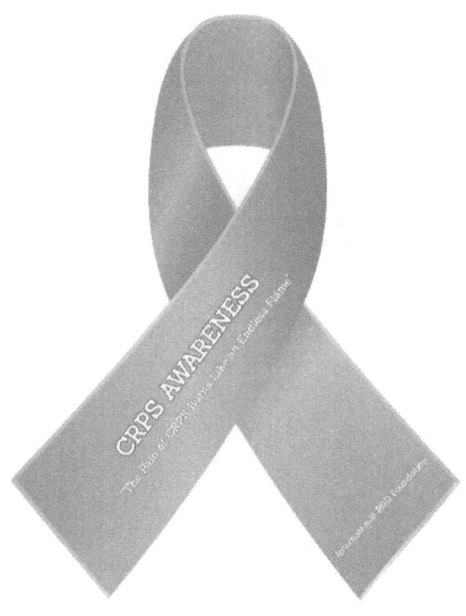

CRPS INFORMATION

For more information about CRPS please visit:

THE INTERNATATIONAL RSD FOUNDATION

www.rsdinfo.com

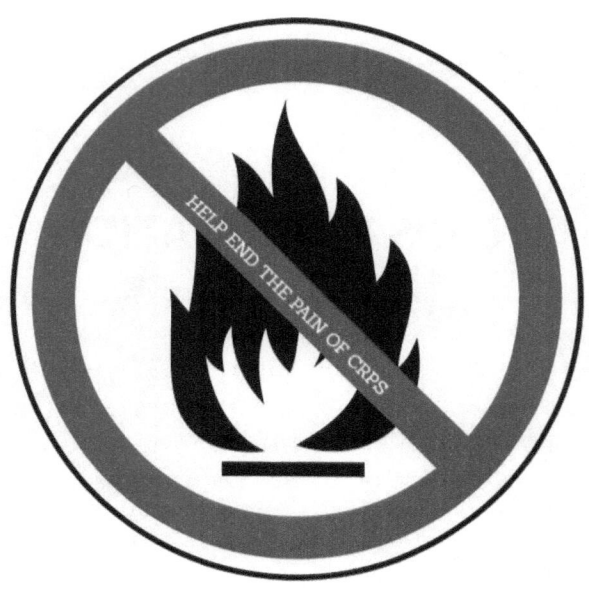

www.ingramcontent.com/pod-product-compliance
Lightning Source LLC
Chambersburg PA
CBHW031549210526
45464CB00003B/1218